Distribution, publication, and copying in any form are prohibited and subject to damages.

TEN HYPNOSES

Copying, publishing, and sharing with third parties are only permitted with the written consent of the author. Please observe the notes on copyright and usage.

Distribution, publication, and copying in any form are prohibited and subject to damages.

Copying, publishing, and sharing with third parties are only permitted with the written consent of the author. Please observe the notes on copyright and usage.

Distribution, publication, and copying in any form are prohibited and subject to damages.

Ingo Michael Simon

TEN HYPNOSES

9

Self-Confidence and Decision-Making

Copying, publishing, and sharing with third parties are only permitted with the written consent of the author. Please observe the notes on copyright and usage.

Distribution, publication, and copying in any form are prohibited and subject to damages.

© 2024 Ingo Michael Simon
All rights reserved.
Independently published
www.ingosimon.com

Important Notes for Urgent Attention:
The contents of this book are based on the practical experiences of the author with hypnosis applications and psychotherapy in a trance state. Although the author has strived for the utmost care, errors or misunderstandings in the presentation cannot be completely excluded. Therapeutic work with people and the application of hypnosis are solely the responsibility of the hypnotist. It cannot be ruled out that parts of this book may be misunderstood or that the application of a presented procedure may cause an undesirable reaction in the client. The author also assumes no co-responsibility if work with a client is carried out with reference to the statements in this book.

The Author:
Ingo Michael Simon studied psychology and education and is a hypnotherapist with practices in southwestern Germany and Switzerland. With the help of hypnosis-supported psychotherapy, he primarily treats people with persistent psychological conditions. His practice focuses on anxiety disorders, pathological compulsions, and psychosomatic illnesses. His therapeutic offerings mainly include classical and modern hypnosis applications and the dreamland therapy he developed himself.

Copying, publishing, and sharing with third parties are only permitted with the written consent of the author. Please observe the notes on copyright and usage.

Notes on Copyright and Usage

Copying, publishing, and sharing with third parties is prohibited and only permitted with the written consent of the author. Please observe the following copyright and usage guidelines.

This work has been carefully crafted and created to the best of the author's knowledge and personal experience. It comprises text templates and application guidelines for professional hypnosis sessions. The author is a licensed psychotherapist with extensive experience in psychotherapy, coaching, and personal training using hypnotic techniques and methods. Nevertheless, the author and the publisher assume no liability for the accuracy of information, instructions, and advice, nor for any typographical errors. The author and publisher accept no responsibility or liability for the application of these texts and recommendations with clients or patients, nor for any potential consequences or unexpected reactions. It is expressly noted that the application of therapeutic and advisory techniques and formulations lies solely and entirely within the responsibility of the practitioner. This also applies to adherence to the boundaries of legally regulated medical and therapeutic practices. The fact that a book containing action proposals is freely available for sale does not imply that its application with clients or patients is permitted for everyone.

Distribution, publication, and copying in any form are prohibited and subject to damages.

Copying, publishing, and sharing with third parties are only permitted with the written consent of the author. Please observe the notes on copyright and usage.

Distribution, publication, and copying in any form are prohibited and subject to damages.

Table of contents

Introduction 9

#1 11

#2 16

#3 21

#4 26

#5 32

#6 37

#7 42

#8 48

#9 53

#10 58

Overview of All Titles in the Series "Ten Hypnoses" 63

Copying, publishing, and sharing with third parties are only permitted with the written consent of the author. Please observe the notes on copyright and usage.

Distribution, publication, and copying in any form are prohibited and subject to damages.

Copying, publishing, and sharing with third parties are only permitted with the written consent of the author. Please observe the notes on copyright and usage.

Introduction

The series "Ten Hypnoses" is very well known in Germany, Austria, and Switzerland as a collection of texts for therapeutic work and is used by numerous psychotherapeutic practices, doctors, therapists, coaches, and other helping professionals. I am pleased to now be able to offer these texts in other countries as well.

Most therapists have their own methods for inducing and deepening trance as well as for exiting trance. Therefore, I have focused on the main part of the hypnosis. The texts in this book can be integrated as the main part into any hypnosis process.

The texts in this collection use various hypnosis techniques. I will not explain these in detail, as I assume that users have the appropriate training. It is also not necessary to understand the exact structure or functioning of the different parts. The texts can simply be read aloud, and they will have their effect.

Decide for yourself which text best suits your client or patient at any given time. You can also combine passages from different texts. It is not about using all ten hypnoses in sequence. It is a selection of possibilities.

I want to emphasize that books cannot replace therapy. Psychotherapy or other therapeutic treatments involve much more. A careful diagnosis is the necessary basis for deciding on the use of methods, including whether hypnosis or one of my texts should be used. Even in this case, preparatory discussions, follow-up discussions during the session, and of course, a therapeutic concept for the sequence of sessions and the content approaches are essential parts of therapy. This cannot and should not be achieved with a collection of texts.

In any case, I wish you much success in your work and I am pleased if my text templates can contribute in a small way.

Ingo Michael Simon

#1

You have decided that it is now time to be open and sociable... ... You want to approach other people with a sense of security and pride and feel good about it... ... You have a very clear idea of what you want, and you know exactly what you want... ... You want to meet other people with curiosity and have a good and secure feeling... ... That is your goal... ... It is truly remarkable that you have made a firm decision deep within you to achieve this goal now... ... The good news is: you can achieve this goal today... ... on this very day... ... and faster than you think... ... The path to this goal lies within you... ... and you will find it here and now... ... Isn't it amazing how clear this becomes to you at this moment? ... ... really remarkable how well you manage to have this inner clarity right now... ... This is the best prerequisite to turn this inner clarity into an external truth now... ... Clarity and truth... ...

So you begin to focus your strength... ... All the energy in your body flows into your legs... ... The more you manage to focus your attention on your legs and concentrate entirely on the feeling in your legs, the stronger they actually become... ... so strong that they enable you to walk powerfully... ... It is truly amazing how helpful a powerful walk, a good and strong feeling can be... ... You see yourself in your mind's eye walking through a crowd of people with strong and broad steps... ... upright and strong... ... carried by your own strength... ... Steady and unshakeable, you stride on both legs... ... full of self-confidence... ... secure and strong... ... secure and strong... ... Your walk becomes more forceful... ... Nothing could stop you... ... The more you manage to focus your attention on your legs and concentrate entirely on the feeling in your legs, the better you succeed in imagining your self-confidence in the crowd... ... and simultaneously clarity becomes truth... ... and simultaneously clarity becomes truth... ... Isn't it amazing how easy this can be... ...

Now focus your attention on your arms... ... Then you feel the strength in your arms... ... They are strong and powerful... ... Your shoulders are also stable and strong... ... So your inner strength becomes greater and your self-confidence more apparent... ... A strong posture gives you strength and self-confidence... ... The more you manage to focus your attention on your shoulders and arms and concentrate entirely on the feeling in your arms, the stronger they actually become... ... and simultaneously clarity becomes truth... ... and simultaneously clarity becomes truth... ... Isn't it amazing how easy this can be... ...

You breathe freely in and out... ... just like now... ... You breathe deeply and feel your own strength more and more... ... Strength in your walk... ... Strength in your posture... ... Strength in your thoughts... ... Your gaze is firm and determined... ... Your face relaxes, and you feel comfortable... ... You breathe deeply and feel good in this strength... ... People walk past you... ... You meet them openly and freely... ... You make friendly contact with them... ... You feel your strength... ... You let all these people walk past you... ... Steady and stable, you stand among all the people and feel comfortable... ... But you can do much more... ... You want much more... ... You find a friendly person and simply start a conversation... ... You have a short chat with them as you walk by... ... You are happy to be so uninhibited and relaxed... ... You don't think at all about what others might think... ... The thoughts of others no longer matter to you... ... Only your own well-being matters... ... which becomes stronger and stronger... ... You look into the faces of the people walking past you... ... You sense how restless they are and at the same time feel your own calmness and strength... ... Everything is much easier when you continue walking with a powerful and forward-directed stride... ... just like now... ... just like now... ... It's easy for you to be in the crowd and even look people in the face... ... and you yourself decide when to stop and speak to someone... ... to feel that you can use your strength optimally then... ... and indeed you can... ... Just as you can move forward with a firm step, so you can also strongly and enthusiastically make contact with other people and have an interesting conversation... ...

Today you imagine this very clearly, as if you could watch yourself in a huge mirror talking to other people... ... You watch yourself and are amazed at how well you can actually do it when you focus on your own strength... ...

The more you manage to feel your own strength and imagine it, the better you will be able to overcome yourself and approach people... ...

So now you focus on the idea of strength... ... the strength that shows in your body... ... in your posture... ... in your steady walk... ... and at the same time, your ability to approach people and feel good about it becomes stronger and stronger... ... You see possible rejections as unimportant... ... It doesn't matter at all if someone rejects you because you know that person wasn't the right one... ... You know that you are still an interesting person, and you will find someone else who recognizes that and is truly interested in you... ...

Your inner truth today, at this very moment, is that you are strong... ... confident... ... secure and sovereign... ... You have observed yourself in your mind's eye and have today turned your inner clarity into external truth... ... You can do this every day... ... You have looked at yourself as if in a mirror... ... So just turn your inner mirror into external truth as well... ... Every glance in a mirror should from now on remind you that you already have this strength and self-confidence... ... and immediately it becomes an external truth... ... just like now... ... just like now...

#2

You have resolved to be open and sociable again from today... ... You have a good plan and you also know what you want... ... To meet people around you with self-confidence and interest and be strong while doing so... ... strong and calm, quite naturally... ... That is your goal... ... Today you can achieve this goal... ... faster than you think... ... The solution to your former insecurity lies deep within you... ... Today you find this solution and can change everything... ... You have already internally prepared to change everything today... ... it is truly admirable how well you have managed this and how quickly you can actually bring about changes now... ... how quickly and well you can now really achieve your goal... ...

... ... You start by focusing your strength... ... All the energy in your body flows into your legs... ... They provide a firm stand... ... It is truly amazing how important strong legs are for a good and strong feeling... ... You see yourself standing on both legs... ... upright and strong... ... carried by your own strength... ... Steady and unshakeable, you stand on both legs... ... Your stand becomes firmer... ... Nothing could shake you... ... Then you feel the strength in your arms... ... They are strong and powerful... ... Your shoulders are also stable and strong... ... So your inner strength becomes greater, your self-confidence more apparent... ...

... ... You breathe freely in and out... ... just like now... ... You breathe deeply and feel your own strength more and more... ... Strength in your legs... ... Strength in your arms... ... Strength in your shoulders... ... You stand as secure as a tree... ... You feel your own strength, which becomes stronger and stronger... ... Your head is held high and stable... ... Your gaze is firm and straightforward... ... Your face relaxes, and you feel comfortable... ... You breathe deeply and feel good in this strength... ... People walk past you... ... You smile at them and wave... ... You make friendly contact with them... ... You feel your strength... ... You let all these people walk past you... ... Steady and stable, you stand among all the people and feel comfortable... ... But you can do more... ... You want more... ... You find a friendly person and simply greet them... ... You wish them a good day and move on... ... You are happy to be so uninhibited and relaxed... ... You don't think at all about what others might think... ... The thoughts of others no longer matter to you... ... Only your own strength matters... ... which becomes stronger and stronger... ... You look into the faces of the people walking past you... ... You sense how restless they are and feel your own calmness and strength... ... Everything is much easier when you stand upright with powerful legs... with strong arms and broad shoulders... ... with your head held high... ... just like now... ... just like now... ... It's easy for you to stand in the crowd and even look people in the face... ... Every time you look someone in the face, you feel the strength in your legs... ... Every time you look someone in the face, you feel the strength in your arms... ... Every time you look someone in the face, you feel the strength in your shoulders... ... Every time you look someone in the face, you feel your head held high... ... Every time you look someone in the face, you feel your firm gaze... ...

... ... You want even more... ... You want to be even stronger... ... You want to look people in the eyes and feel good... ... You want to feel free... ... You want to feel strong... ... just like now... ... You want to approach interesting people and talk to them... ... uninhibited and relaxed... ... quite naturally... ... So you try it out, and it spontaneously works... ... much easier than you thought... ... You look directly into the eyes of some people who walk past you and let them move on... ... You feel strong and stable doing so... ... Your legs support you... ... They are firm and strong... ... Your arms remain strong

... ... Your shoulders are broad and becoming broader and stronger... ... Your head is straight, and your gaze is firm... ...

... ... It is truly amazing how easy it is for you today... ... how quickly you can achieve your goals... ... now and every other day... ... now and every other day... ...

... ... Then you greet everyone who walks past you very friendly and with a welcoming look... ... You greet every person... ... With each person you greet, your gaze becomes firmer and stronger, and you feel good... ... With each breath, you feel freer and lighter... ... You greet everyone and feel free... ... Some stop briefly and have a conversation with you, and everything is fine... ... You feel free and strong because you have achieved this... ... You can do it, and you feel freer every day... ...

Just like now, it can always be... ... You look people in the face and feel the strength in your legs and arms... ... in your shoulders and head... ... You talk to people and feel courage and strength... ... You feel liberated and can breathe deeply... ... You can breathe freely... ... free and calm... ... The longer you look people in the face and in the eyes, the more confident you become... ... The more you focus on people's eyes, the more you feel your strength... ... now and every other day just like this... ... now and every other day just like this... ...

You remind yourself once again that every inner truth can become external truth... ... Everything you can think and imagine can immediately become truth if you want it that way... ... So you want it with all your strength... ... to meet people with pride and self-confidence... ... That is your goal... ... Today you have achieved it... ... So you achieve it every day because whenever you look someone in the face, you immediately feel this strength and power again, just like now... ... The more directly you look people in the face, the better and stronger you feel... ... Today and every other day... ... today and every other day...

#3

The following variant of a main part of hypnosis works with an anchor in the form of a handy note with the words "Calmness and Pride" printed on it. An anchor is a trigger that is meant to evoke a certain feeling or thought. We want to help the client use a "reminder card" to quickly adjust to releasing any arising fear in situations where they are the center of attention. We discuss this with the client before the session and prepare the reminder card. This can be a written business card or something similar. The card is prepared and given to the client to hold loosely in their hand or place on their body during hypnosis, for example, on the solar plexus. They should carry the card with them after the hypnosis session, in their pants pocket or jacket pocket.

You often find yourself in the spotlight, being observed by others... ... You often have this fear, this stage fright before your performance... ... You aim to finally put this fear behind you... ... to send it to the place of memories and leave it there... ... because that's where the past belongs... ... You can recall past experiences and feelings of insecurity and fear, but they should not intrude on the present... ... because the present belongs only to you... ... It is important that we only hold onto the past as long as necessary to process and understand what happened... ... You have now reached that point... ... You have processed and understood... ... Therefore, now is the right time to let go... ... to let go of the fear, to let go of the stage fright and send it to the place of memory... ...

... ... You have decided that you want to build calmness and pride to handle your tasks confidently and well... ... to enjoy your performances... ... You have understood that it is up to you to make truth out of your intentions... ... You know that it is you who makes your success... ... and you are ready for it... ... You are ready to give everything necessary to become inwardly calm and proud... ... free from old burdens of the past... ... You have the potential for it... ... you have the strength you need... ...

But you want more... ... You want to be able to fully access your qualities and abilities at any time... ... You want to quickly and completely adopt a calm and proud attitude...

... especially when you might feel nervous again and suddenly notice it... ...

You know the important words, the crucial ones... ... Calmness and pride... ... It's like a message to yourself... ... Calmness and pride... ... It's like a new memory... ... Calmness and pride... ... like an instruction only you can give yourself... ... Calmness and pride... ... Calmness and pride... ...

You have this card with exactly these words on it, the card states your goal... ... Calmness and pride... ... You now feel this inner strength growing stronger within you... ... You know you can achieve everything... ... your will and readiness grow with every breath, and with every breath, it becomes clearer... ... Calmness and pride... ... The card shows you this every day... ... It shows you your task that you can always carry with you... ... Calmness and pride... ... It helps you become stronger every day and eventually always be free... ... As soon as the slightest doubt arises in you, you immediately take the card in your hand and read the words clearly, you look at it... ... Calmness and pride... ... Then you immediately feel the effect, you feel that this is your truth... ... You do this every day... ... ... You simply let go of the fear... ... You simply let go of the fear... ...

The card shows you this every day... It shows you your own attitude that you can always carry with you... ... It helps you through difficult moments... ... As soon as the slightest doubt arises in you, you immediately take the card in your hand and look at it... ... Calmness and pride... ... Then you immediately feel the effect, you feel that this is your truth... ...

... ... Take your reminder card consciously in your hand now... ... Hold it firmly... ... Have you noticed that you are holding onto something again?... ... This time you are holding onto calmness and pride... ... That's a good hold... ... holding onto your goal of calmness and pride... ... holding onto the fact that you are important to yourself... ... holding onto your goal to free yourself... ... holding onto the fact that nothing is more important to you than calmness and pride... ... holding onto only calmness and pride... ... holding onto only calmness and pride... ... The card you feel between your fingers reminds you of this... ... it helps you release the fear... ... it helps you be free and take new paths... ... free and open with calmness and pride towards the future... ... free and open... ... every day...

... ... [Ask the client now to open their eyes and read the word in trance. This enhances the effect. Opening the eyes is a fractionation, which can be done without special announcement or counting. Everyone can open their eyes in trance. In a stable and deep trance, it's a bit cumbersome because the client is tired and sluggish. Just stick with suggestive encouragement until the eyes open and the card is read.] ...

... ... Consciously feel the reminder card between your fingers now, and if you want, briefly open your eyes and look at the card... ... open your eyes and read what is written there... ... Calmness and pride... ... Calmness and pride... ... Now close your eyes again and let the read words sink deep within you... ... very deep...

You still feel the card between your fingers... ... You know it can remind you every day to be free by letting go of the fear and building calmness and pride... ... Whenever you take the card in your hand and read it, you immediately feel that you become inwardly freer and calmer... ... freer and calmer... ... Whenever you carry the card with you, you feel inwardly calmer and freer... ... Calmness and pride... ... This happens automatically because your inner self knows that this card reminds you of what you did today... ... your own liberation...

#4

The following hypnosis session works with an acoustic anchor. An anchor is a trigger that is meant to evoke a certain feeling or thought. We want to help the client evoke the feeling of self-confidence within them using a reproducible sound. In the state of trance, the feeling of self-confidence is initially emphasized through suggestions. Then a sound is presented and associated with this feeling (anchored). This can be any sound that is deliberately and controllably presented. In the era of ubiquitous smartphones or cell phones, an alarm ring tone can be used. The client can easily ensure that they hear this sound several times a day. They just need to set the alarm. It's a good idea to use the same tone for incoming messages (SMS, emails, etc.). A frequent smartphone user will then often hear their anchor. Make sure during the session that you can control the tone to be used without the client's phone actually ringing due to an incoming call or message. Call forwarding should be set up for the duration of the session. Of course, this only works if your client trusts you with their phone. A new tone should be used so that it is not already emotionally charged. You can also generally suggest and anchor "any sound your phone makes..." but try it with the ring tone. Many clients are enthusiastic about phone hypnosis. And – it works excellently!

Being strong is your goal... ... You have firmly resolved to take your life into your own hands and always find the strength within you to assert yourself and push through... ... to overcome your insecurity and fear of rejection again and again... ... to find self-determination in your life again... ... to pursue goals worth fighting for... ... to achieve your goals and your satisfaction... ... From now on, you will succeed... ... because you are now on the path to becoming truly self-confident and strong... ... This thought is so strong that today you fully commit yourself to feeling exactly that way, self-confident and strong... ...

... ... Today we are working with an anchor, you already know that... ... and you also know that your phone will be the anchor... ... Perhaps you are already wondering how quickly this anchor will work... ... how soon it might happen that a ring tone on your phone immediately gives you a feeling of self-confidence and courage... ... It might surprise you how well this anchor works... ... how quickly you actually get into this feeling of self-confidence and courage, especially when things get tough... ...

... ... Today is the first day of your new life... ... a life where you manage to quickly get into a feeling of self-confidence and courage again and again... ... The good thing is, it is much easier than you thought... ... Perhaps you wonder how you can best and quickest feel self-confidence and courage... ...

... ... It is easier than you thought... ... For this, you now mentally go back to a time when you felt really good, really strong and full of self-confidence, because you have had such a time before... ... maybe to the best time of your life... ... maybe it was a long period, a few years... ... or maybe there was a short time when you felt really strong... ... maybe just a very brief moment, but it was so intense that you can remember it now... ... If you want, just take a very intense fantasy of how it could be once you are really strong and courageous... ... Imagine how you naturally do what you've always wanted to do... ... A beautiful feeling of courage and strength... ... and go completely into this feeling... ... feel how good it is... ... The more you focus on your memory or your fantasy, the more intensely you can feel the good life feeling... .... maybe freedom... ... lightness... ... joy... ... happiness... ... strength and courage... ... strength and courage... ... You feel really good in this memory... ... or in this fantasy... ... You feel better and better... ... The more you focus on your memory or your fantasy, the more intensely you can feel the self-confidence within you... ... just like that... ... Let the feeling in you become more and more beautiful... ... This is exactly the feeling you need... ... This is exactly the feeling you need every day... ...

... ... You can secure it... ... You can now ensure that this also works for you in your waking everyday life... ... just like now... ... every day just like now... ... It is very simple... ... You can go into this feeling every day and then feel good... ... You can do it again and again, especially when things get tough... ... Then it suddenly becomes easy to feel the good life feeling... ... Then it suddenly becomes easy to choose life... ...

...... [Prepare the phone now. Make sure you can also retrieve the desired tone without searching or trying.] ...

Now concentrate and wait for the ring tone you will hear soon because this ring tone connects with the strong feeling of self-confidence and makes it even stronger......

...... [Let the phone ring now] ...... There it is, that's your signal of self-confidence, courage, and strength...... This ring tone is the most important sound for you......

...... [Let the phone ring now] ...... This ring tone strengthens your courage......

...... [Let the phone ring now] ...... This ring tone awakens your self-confidence......

...... [Let the phone ring now] ...... This ring tone makes you braver with each time......

...... [Let the phone ring now] ...... Whenever you hear this ring tone, you feel your courage......

...... And whenever you hear this specific ring tone, you immediately feel strong and stronger...... Whenever you perceive exactly this tone, you feel clearly that you are self-confident and that your courage increases with each ring...

… Even when you just think about the ring tone or take your phone in your hand, you can already feel that you are strong… …

Whenever you hear the ring tone, the feeling of strength immediately awakens in you, you immediately feel self-confident and strong… … and if you want to intensify the feeling or urgently need it – Just let your phone ring, just like now… … [Let the phone ring now] … … just like now… … [Let the phone ring now] … … [Let the phone ring now] … …

#5

You are faced with a difficult decision and want to find the right resolution today... ... You have decided that it is now time to make the upcoming decision... ... You already have all the necessary information, so you can find your decision today... ... It is good that you now want to make up your mind... ... You want to gain more clarity, perhaps take the last step... ... and then commit yourself... ...

You now reconsider the options you have and find the two between which you most want to decide... ... You visualize both options as headlines... ... You come up with a suitable headline for the first option, like a headline in a newspaper, and imagine a large white poster with this headline on it... ... Formulate your inner headline at your own pace... ... in your own time... ... Then write it in big, bold letters on the white poster... ... Look at it closely... ... Read it and let the words sink in... ... perhaps it is just a single word of the decision that forms your headline... ... Look closely and consciously perceive the headline... ... Pay attention to the feeling it evokes in you and let it resonate... ...

... ... [Pause for about half a minute to let the decision option become more emotionally tangible, then continue reading] ... ...

Then you think of a headline for the second option... ... Take your time with it too... ... in your own pace... ... in your own time... ... and also imagine a large white poster with this headline on it... ... Look at it closely... ... Read it and let the words sink in... ... perhaps it is just a single word of the decision that forms your headline... ... Look closely and consciously perceive the headline... ... Pay attention to the feeling it evokes in you and let it resonate... ...

... ... [Pause for about half a minute to let the decision option become more emotionally tangible, then continue reading] ... ...

So now you have both options before your eyes... ... You have thought about both options many times, considering which one is the best... ... Deep down, you already know how you want to decide... ...

You have hesitated because you have thought about many things... ... about the demands of others... ... perhaps about this inner urge to fulfill something, but today you only need to fulfill something for yourself, to be there for yourself... ... It is about you and your decision... ... about you and your decision... ... So you make clear to yourself once again what is really important to you... ... what you want... ... what you need to make a good decision for yourself... ... what is really good for you... ... Others are now unimportant... ... Others make their own decisions, but you make your decision today... ... For this, your feeling is important... ... Therefore, you now focus entirely on your body feeling... ... You know that the gut usually decides... ... So pay attention to your gut feeling... ... Feel how your gut feels... ... Feel how your body feels... ...

Then look at the poster with the first option... ... Read the headline of the possible decision again and now feel your gut feeling... ... Pay attention only to the feeling... ... Perceive it clearly... ... your gut feeling... ... Let go of all thoughts, now it is only about the gut feeling... ... good, like that... ... focus entirely on it and feel the feeling, whatever it may be... ... Now look at the second poster... ... Look at this headline of the possible decision too and immediately feel into your gut... ... Let the feeling become clear... ... Let go of all thoughts and go entirely into the gut feeling... ... good, like that... ... focus entirely on it and feel the feeling, whatever it may be... ...

Now take a deep breath... ... Allow yourself to relax... ... and calm down... ... and pay attention to the decision your gut has shown you... ... Your gut has already shown you with which headline you feel better, which feels right... ... You can repeat it... ... Just look alternately at both posters and ask your gut what it feels... ...

You sense your inner decision... ... You make clear to yourself that only the decision your gut feels is right is the right one... ... You allow yourself to listen to your gut, which does not need the mind, which always makes accurate decisions for you if you just allow it to send you signals... ... You feel which decision is right for you... ... and you allow yourself to decide just as your gut does... ... just like that... ... Put the wrong poster aside and look only at the poster with the good headline... ... Let your gut feeling intensively resonate, let it show you that your decision is good because it is your decision... ...

You now know exactly what matters to you... ... You know your decision and resolve to stick with it... ... To maintain your inner security, you can write a poster with your decision and place it somewhere you can often see it... ... Think of such a place... ... At the same time, such a place arises within you... ... So you can look at the poster every day... ... externally and within you... ... and each time it reminds you that your decision is good and right... ... and that you are entitled to act according to your own decision... ...

#6

Today, you are preparing for your special performance... ... for your presentation... ... Whenever we stand in front and all eyes are on us, it is about presenting ourselves... ... during lectures... ... at promotional events... ... at the information desk... ... or on the acting stage... ... It is always the same... ... It's about presentation... ... being seen... ... being heard... ... a special occasion where everyone pays attention to us... ... In the past, this has been challenging for you... ... You are familiar with the notion of not being enough... ... not meeting expectations... ... But today, you can do something very special... ... Today, you can prepare... ... prepare so well that you can meet all expectations... ... especially your own, which are higher than those of your audience... ... You know that good preparation is particularly important... ... You have already prepared your content and presentation tools... ... But today, it's about the inner preparation, because that is especially important... ... Today's preparation helps you truly access what you have to offer... ... to access your expertise... ... to access your experience... ... to access your personality and charisma...

You pack your presentation suitcase for this... ... your very own presentation suitcase... ... It lies before you, a sturdy case that protects its contents well, so you can access whatever you need from it at any time... ... Choose the sturdiest suitcase you can imagine... ... maybe made of strong plastic... ... or aluminum... ... choose it to be as stable as it seems to you...

Now open the suitcase... ... It is completely empty... ... You will start filling it soon... ... with your own abilities, with your potential... ... with all your experience... ... your know-how... ... maybe with your tips and tricks for a successful presentation or a deal that might result from it... ... You will pack five special items into your suitcase...

Choose an Item or symbol for your expertise... ... Knowledge is power... ... Knowledge creates an advantage... ... Your knowledge is a key to success... ... Truly amazing how much expertise you actually possess... ... Decide now on an item that represents this expertise... ... Place this item in the suitcase... ... Once you close and take the suitcase with you, your expertise will always be fully and quickly available to you... ...

Now choose an item or symbol for your experience... ... Experience provides security... ... Experience means flexibility... ... Your experience is a key to success... ... Truly amazing how much experience you actually possess... ... Decide now on an item that represents this experience... ... Place this item in the suitcase... ... Once you close and take the suitcase with you, your experience will always be fully and quickly available to you... ...

Next, choose an item or symbol for your charisma... ... Charisma is the radiance of a winner... ... Charisma captivates listeners... ... Your charisma is a key to success... ... Truly amazing how much charisma you actually possess... ... Decide now on an item that represents this charisma... ... Place this item in the suitcase... ... Once you close and take the suitcase with you, your charisma will always be fully and quickly available to you... ...

Now choose an item or symbol for your oratory skills... ... Oratory is the special talent that counts... ... Oratory draws listeners into your spell and convinces them... ... Your oratory skills are a key to success... ... Truly amazing how much oratory skills you actually possess... ... Decide now on an item that represents these oratory skills... ... Place this item in the suitcase... ... Once you close and take the suitcase with you, your oratory skills will always be fully and quickly available to you...

Next, choose an item or symbol for success... ... Success is your goal... ... Success is your goal... ... Quite remarkable how often you have already been successful, how much potential for success you possess... ... Decide now on an item that represents success... ... Place this item in the suitcase... ... Once you close and take the suitcase with you, your success is assured...

As soon as you start your presentation, your suitcase opens by itself and immediately provides you with all these good qualities... ... Expertise... ... Experience... ... Charisma... ... Oratory skills... ... and Success...

Maybe you want even more... ... Well, nothing could be easier... ... Take a suitcase with you to your presentation... ... maybe you already have one with you... ... Open it briefly just before you start, just before your presentation begins...

... Then, open your suitcase briefly, just for yourself, and immediately your inner self provides you with your qualities... ... ... Expertise... ... Experience... ... Charisma... ... Oratory skills... ... and Success...

#7

The following hypnosis session works with the classic arm levitation (floating arm). With the help of suggestions or images, the impression is conveyed during arm levitation that the client's body can move without their conscious effort. The required muscle contraction is carried out "unconsciously" – somewhat inaccurately but understandably expressed: the client's unconscious performs the movement, which the client experiences as being externally controlled. Levitation increases belief in the special effect of hypnosis and shows the client that there is more than what they actively decide and consciously and willingly influence. It is important for the client to be able to observe the floating and then cataleptic (rigid) arm with their own eyes. Therefore, always have the client open their eyes during arm levitations and catalepsies to observe the result. Many clients otherwise believe that the entire arm movement was just a sensory illusion; some do not feel the movement very clearly with closed eyes. Do not worry, opening the eyes does not lose the trance, and the catalepsy remains stable! The *stronger a person's belief in the unconscious power of their organism is, the more positive the changes will be, both in behavioral and emotional changes as well as in the treatment of illnesses. Of course, hypnosis is not a miracle cure. Therefore, never promise a specific success (which, by the way, is prohibited for all therapists anyway).*

You want to feel confident in dealing with other people... ... You want to be stronger and assert yourself... ... You want to finally trust your own abilities and strengths... ... You have decided to be self-confident and sovereign from now on... ... self-confident and sovereign...

Your unconscious helps you with this, and it is probably easier than you think... ... Your unconscious can mobilize your own abilities because everything you have been looking for is already within you... ... You find everything within yourself, exactly today and exactly in this moment... ... Perhaps you are wondering how best to feel that you have the strength and self-confidence within you and can actually use it... ... The good thing is that your unconscious can show you that your self-confidence grows with every word I say...

... You are mentally preparing for your self-confidence to grow a bit each time I say "Trust yourself!"... ... But your unconscious can do even more... ... Because with each step it takes for you, with each step of strengthening your self-confidence, your unconscious lifts your right arm a bit... ... You just have to allow it... ... Whenever I say "Trust yourself," your unconscious lifts your arm a bit and holds it up, it goes very easily and as if by itself, and you realize how much self-confidence has already been built up...

Levitation Phase

It is truly amazing that your unconscious can lift your arm... ... It works... ... Your arm becomes very light whenever I say: Trust yourself... ... Start now... ... Trust yourself... ... Trust yourself... ... Your unconscious helps you and lifts your arm... ... Just allow it and feel your arm move... ... Trust yourself... ... It is truly amazing that your arm is lifted as if by itself... ... Trust yourself... ... and further... ... Trust yourself... ... Trust yourself... ... Your unconscious lifts your arm higher and higher... ... Trust yourself and higher... ... Trust yourself and higher... ... Just like that... ... Trust yourself... ... good... ... Trust yourself... ... good...

[Now keep at it and repeat the formula "Trust yourself" and observe the arm. If it is lifted step by step, simply repeat the suggestion. If the arm does not cooperate immediately, support it a bit with auxiliary suggestions like "Your unconscious helps you and lifts your arm now. Allow it."]

Catalepsy Phase

Your arm is as light as a feather and at the same time very firm... ... as firm as your self-confidence... ... Your arm now becomes very firm and rigid... ... Your unconscious holds your arm in exactly this position... ... just like that... ... Your arm becomes firmer, completely immovable... ... Nothing and no one can move your arm now... ... Your arm is rigid like an iron rod... ... Your self-confidence is now as strong and firm as your arm... ... and just as light... ... Your arm is firm, and just as firm is your self-confidence now... ... Your arm shows it to you... ... It is very firm and remains in exactly this position...

Fractionation Phase

... ... You can look at it... ... When I tell you to open your eyes, you can simply open your eyes and observe your arm, which remains held as if by itself... ... When I then tell you to close your eyes again, you simply do so, and your self-confidence will grow even more... ... Just open your eyes, and your arm remains firm and stable in exactly this position... ... firm and stable... ... Open your eyes and look at your arm...

[Stay at it and insist that the client opens their eyes and observes their arm. Do not worry, the catalepsy remains! If in doubt, support with suggestions like "Your arm remains just like this... Your arm continues to float in the air..."]

And now close your eyes again, and your self-confidence grows even stronger and more stable... ... You become stronger and stronger...

Your arm now becomes movable again and

slowly sinks back to the surface, your self-confidence being deeply anchored in the process... ... and as soon as your arm touches the surface, your great self-confidence is deeply anchored in you and is available to you at any time... ... Your arm sinks back to the surface, and your self-confidence is deeply anchored...

[Stay with suggestions until the arm actually reaches the surface "Your arm becomes movable and sinks down"… "Your arm becomes heavy and sinks to the surface"…]

Your arm is now completely movable and under your control. Move your arm and hand and check that you indeed have full control over your body!

#8

You want to feel confident in dealing with other people... ... You want to be stronger and assert yourself... ... You want to finally trust your own abilities and strengths... ... You have decided to be self-confident and sovereign from now on... ... self-confident and sovereign... ... You know many self-confident people and many strong personalities... ... They appear great to you... ... You perceive them as impressive and strong... ... Then you think it should be possible to be just as strong and great... ... and indeed you can be, because today you find this greatness and strength within you... ... Today you are great... ... Today you are strong...

... ... Breathe deeply and expand your chest... ... The deep inhalation frees you... ... It opens up a space for you... ... So breathe deeply again... ... [in the client's breathing rhythm please]... ... breathe deeply... ... good... ... Continue... ... Breathe deeply and fully... ...

… … Isn't it wonderfully freeing to breathe so deeply and spread yourself out… … You spread out at your own pace… … This space here is only for you…

… … [Now please ensure that breathing continues intensely and always speak the following suggestions with a deep inhalation of the client. Of course, the client can simply keep breathing. Just wait with the crucial suggestions until the next breath. Timing is important! If the text says "Client inhales," that should be the case. If they are exhaling, simply wait for the next breath.]…

… … [Client inhales]… Breathe deeply and fully and fill the room with your personality… … [Client inhales]… Your aura radiates in all directions… … You now have this special charisma that can fascinate others… … again… … [Client inhales]… Fill the room with your personality… … good…

… … [Client inhales]… Breathe deeply and fully and fill the room with your thoughts… … In all directions, you extend your thoughts… … You grow larger with each thought you send into the room… … Isn't it pleasant to have so much space for once… … again… … [Client inhales]… Fill the room with your thoughts… … good…

... ... [Client inhales]... Breathe deeply and fully and fill the room with your decisions... ... In all directions, you extend your will... ... You grow larger with each demand you send into the room... ... Isn't it pleasant to have so much space for your will and demands... ... again... ... [Client inhales]... Fill the room with your decisions... ... good...

... ... You allow yourself here and now to fill the room only with yourself... ... You feel how great you are... ... You even become larger... ... It is like growing... ... You are like a plant that grows and thrives... ... stretches and reaches toward the sun... ... So you also stretch and reach inwardly and become larger and stronger... ... A deep power within you makes its way outside... ... You can feel it... ... You are much larger than you thought... ... Imagine yourself standing among many people... ... Hundreds of people stand around you... ... With each breath, you become larger, soon towering over everyone... ... Everyone stands around you like dwarfs... ... They look up to you... ... because you are the greatest of all... ... You can feel this greatness and the power that comes from your greatness... ... The more intensely you imagine this picture, the better you can also feel the power within you... ... With each breath, you feel stronger and more courageous... ... You know you can rely on your abilities... ... It is truly amazing how well you manage to feel stronger...

... ... Focus on your feeling... ... Perceive your own strength... ... Let it grow stronger... ... Imagine yourself facing a challenge you were once afraid of... ... You see yourself in a situation that was often difficult for you in the past... ... Today you can take on this challenge... ... You can face it... ... Watch yourself succeeding in overcoming the challenge easily and with a good feeling... ... You see yourself as the winner in the battle with yourself... ... Winner in the battle with your fear and insecurity... ... You feel the good feeling... ... You know how wonderful it is to have mastered the challenge today... ... You can trust that you can always do it again... ... The more intensely you imagine the situation that was once so difficult, the easier it is to feel your own strength now... ... Your trust in your own abilities grows... ... With each breath, your trust in yourself becomes firmer and more stable... ... It is truly amazing how quickly you manage to become so strong... ... to be so strong... ... to stay so strong... ... You trust yourself more and more... ... You let fear bounce off you... ... Fear was yesterday... ...

Today, there is only courage where fear once was... ... Today, there is only strength where there once was a feeling of weakness... ... Today, you trust your own abilities... ... You are a winner...

Every day you can become stronger... ... whenever you want to feel your own strength... ... your assertiveness and self-confidence... ... You simply breathe deeply and fully, making yourself strong again... ... because each deep breath reminds your entire organism that you have this strength... ... that you are allowed and will take up space... ... Whenever you need strength, you breathe deeply and fully, and immediately the self-confidence you feel now is available to you...

#9

You go into the land of dreams... ... In this beautiful land, everything is possible... ... You look around and find the most beautiful natural landscape you can imagine... ... Mountains and valleys... ... Rivers and lakes... ... Meadows and forests... ... And everywhere the plants bloom, and everything grows and thrives... ...

You find a wide path that leads across this land... ... It will be your path today... ... On the paths of the dreamland, you always find yourself... ... You simply follow this wide path... ... Full of trust, you wander along this path through the land of your dreams and approach a forest... ... A forest of tall and old trees... ... You follow the path and enter the forest... ... You feel comfortable and go deeper and deeper into this forest... ... And among the many old trees, there are also smaller ones that are still young... ... even very small trees, tiny shoots that have just emerged... ... This is the forest of your thoughts, and all your thoughts are here... ... They are waiting here for you... ... All the thoughts you have ever thought... ... all the thoughts you will one day think are already here... ... And also, all the thoughts you could have at this very moment are here... ... They are stored here for you...

You are looking for this one special thought that can help you the most today, to change everything you want to change... ... the very special thought, perhaps the spark of an idea... ... or a decision... ... You look deep into the forest and see large stones lying everywhere among the trees... ... They look like stone memorial plaques... ... And that is exactly what they are... ... Plaques that carry your thoughts... ... Many lie in the darkness... ... others are clear and easy to see, as if they are illuminated so that you can see them better... ... On some, you find a word... ... like an engraving... ... others perhaps carry a short sentence... ... or simply a symbol... ... a special sign as a thought of yours... ... Perhaps you even discover a picture on some...

... ... You leave the wide path and walk deeper and deeper into the forest, deeper and deeper into your own thoughts... ... And you see the memorial plaques of your own thoughts over and over again... ... Some light up and show you a thought... ... Others remain in the shadows, and you cannot read anything on them... ... You go deeper into the forest because you are looking for that one thought... ... for the very special thought... ... Today, you want to find the most important thought... ... You want to find the thought that can help you the most right now... ... Today, you can find the special thought... ... The thought that can help you the most, the most important one...

You approach a very large memorial stone... ... It is the largest and most beautiful by far... ... On it, you find the thought of the moment... ... The thought that can help you the most... ... You get closer and closer... ... Through the treetops, a golden ray of light falls and bathes this stone in golden light... ... It lights up, and you recognize the inscription... ... You recognize the thought of the moment... ... You can read it... ... Perhaps you expected this thought, or maybe it surprises you. But whatever it is - It is the most important thought... ... And if you cannot recognize it clearly, that is also completely fine, because the thought is here... ... That is enough... ... Then you simply place both hands on the stone and let the thought flow deep into your feeling and sense it... ... Perhaps now or a little later... ... Let your thought or the feeling that is now there simply work...

… … You turn around and walk back through the trees… … Filled with the most important thought, you return to the wide path… … You trust that this special thought will help you, whatever it is, even if you do not yet know why this thought is so important… … You walk through the trees and notice that the forest is much brighter than before… … much more light floods the forest of your thoughts, and many memorial plaques light up… … You keep walking, let yourself be guided by your feeling, and come back to the wide path and follow it further…

You let the special thought you found today work deep within you and trust that it is truly especially important… … It helps you make every important decision… … This one thought is the special message of your unconscious, the hint for you, what you should pay attention to right now… … Your most important thought…

You reach the edge of the forest and step outside into the sun… … On a beautiful meadow, you find a comfortable place to rest… … You lie down and sink into your thoughts and dreams… … On your skin, you feel the warmth of the sun, which gives you strength and a sense of well-being… … And you feel that the special thought you found spreads within you like a warm breeze... ... Even if it might be an unpleasant thought, it will help you make good decisions and follow a good path... ... It spreads within you to inform every cell of your body about the thought... ... about this inner truth that is so important and significant... ... Then you think about the fact that the land of dreams lies deep within you. It has always been there. I am just telling you about it...

#10

You go into the land of dreams... ... You stand before a signpost that says "To the Place of Decision"... ... The sign stands at a narrow path that leads straight through the land of dreams... ... So you follow this path that takes you to the place of decisions... ... On the way there, you think about how difficult decisions have been in your life... ... You know the situation of having to make many decisions and sometimes not knowing where to start... ... Sometimes it's just a few important decisions to be made, but that can also be very difficult... ... Perhaps it's just one single decision that it's about... ... Sometimes we postpone them because we're afraid of doing something wrong or making a decision that we might regret later... ... and maybe it can't be changed then, has caused so much that it could be too late to reverse everything with a new decision...

... ... You are inwardly in exactly such a situation... ... Maybe you don't know yet how your decision will turn out... ... or you know exactly but struggle with the responsibility that comes with it... ... with the bad conscience or the guilt that might come up... ... You encounter a group of people... ... many of them you know, others you have never seen... ... These are all the people who have tried or are still trying to influence your decision... ... those who expect a specific decision from you... ... all who have demands and expectations of you are here... ... Some you knew would be here because you are familiar with their demands and expectations... ... Perhaps you also meet familiar faces whose presence surprises you... ... They appear before your inner eye because they also have certain expectations... ... Maybe they haven't expressed them or you overheard them... ... But these people have expectations; that's why they show up here... ... Then there are others you don't know because there are many influences on your decisions that you don't immediately feel... ... There are people who affect you because they have demands on others who then build their behavior toward you on that... ... Then there are also people who you encounter but don't have a face... ... They don't show themselves, making their influence felt from the shadows... ... that exists too... ... You look at them... ... You feel all the demands and expectations... ... but you keep walking... ... further to the place of decisions because it's about your decision... ... It's about what you want... ... what you think is right... ... what you ultimately must decide... ... You can't fulfill all demands, and you don't want to either... ... The truth is, you don't have to, because you are not responsible for all those who make demands... ... It suddenly gets dark around you, as if you are walking through a cave... ... It gets darker and quieter, but you can still see the narrow path well and follow it further... ... deeper and deeper into the land of dreams... ... Then it suddenly becomes bright, and you stand on a large round place... ... The ground is covered with sand, and the place is surrounded by a curtain of golden light... ... You stand in the middle of the place; if you want, make yourself comfortable... ... Sit in the soft, warm sand...

... ... The curtain before you slowly opens... ... The curtain of light opens... ... You see a figure coming toward you in the golden light... ... They come closer and step through the curtain... ... It is the person who could comfort you best in your life... ... whoever that may have been... ... This person comes here in the land of dreams, at the place of decisions, to help you with your decision... ... Maybe it's a person who has comforted you many times in your life... ... maybe only a few times or even just once, but so intensely that you can feel this comfort again now... ... this strength that comes from the affection and love of this person and helps you... ... Perhaps you meet here in the land of dreams, at the place of decisions, a person who no longer lives on this earth... ... a person who comforted you in your childhood and has already passed away... ... In the land of dreams, everything is possible... ... here you can meet anyone important to you... ... whether this person still lives in your world or not...

... ... This friendly and good person, your best comforter, or your best comforter comes to you in the middle of the place and hugs you... ... So, they give you comfort and strength even now... ... hope and confidence... ... the strength you need to make your decision or finally stand by it... ... Let the strength and magic that emanates from this person and can help you be there... ... Deep inside, you feel that you also have this strength... ... that you can make your decision... ... that you can represent it and stand by it because it is the right one for you... ... In your deepest self, you have already made your decision... ... Here it becomes clear to you... ... You stand on the place of decision... ... surrounded by golden light... ... accompanied by the person who could and can give you the most hope and comfort... ... today as back then... ... today as back then...

... ... Then you both sit down in the middle of the place, and you enjoy the peace and the support... ... You feel much safer and stronger now... ... You know you can trust in the support and comfort of your helper or helper... ... now at the place of decisions... ... and every day deep inside you... ... because a piece of this helping person lives deep inside you and is always with you... ... whatever happens... ... whatever you experience or do... ... Your inner helper or helper is always with you... ... in the land of dreams... ... in this land that lies deep within you and allows you everything you can dream of... ... Then you think about the fact that the land of dreams is deep inside you. It has always been there. I am just telling you about it...

Distribution, publication, and copying in any form are prohibited and subject to damages.

Overview of All Titles in the Series "Ten Hypnoses"

Volume 1: Smoking Cessation
Volume 2: Anxiety and Restlessness
Volume 3: Burnout
Volume 4: Reducing Overweight
Volume 5: Coping with the Past
Volume 6: Suicidal Thoughts and Attempts
Volume 7: Psycho-Oncology
Volume 8: Obsessions and Tics
Volume 9: Self-Confidence and Decision-Making
Volume 10: Grief Work
Volume 11: Psychosomatics
Volume 12: Chronic Pain
Volume 13: Depressive Thoughts
Volume 14: Panic Attacks
Volume 15: Domestic Violence, Victim Support
Volume 16: Post-Traumatic Stress
Volume 17: Exam Anxiety and Stage Fright
Volume 18: Anti-Violence Training, Offender Support
Volume 19: Addiction Tendencies
Volume 20: Social Phobia and Fear of Contact
Volume 21: Nail Biting
Volume 22: Self-Awareness and Self-Love
Volume 23: Teeth Grinding and Night Clenching
Volume 24: Feelings of Guilt
Volume 25: Fear in Crowds
Volume 26: Fear of Flying, Aviophobia
Volume 27: Fear in Enclosed Spaces, Claustrophobia
Volume 28: Tinnitus, Ear Noises
Volume 29: Fear of Heights
Volume 30: Neurodermatitis

Copying, publishing, and sharing with third parties are only permitted with the written consent of the author. Please observe the notes on copyright and usage.

Volume 31: Finding Inner Balance
Volume 32: Overcoming Loneliness
Volume 33: Fear of Illness, Hypochondria
Volume 34: Anticipatory Anxiety, Fear of Fear
Volume 35: Jealousy in Relationships
Volume 36: Driving Anxiety
Volume 37: New Start after Separation
Volume 38: Fear of Injections
Volume 39: Heart Anxiety Neurosis
Volume 40: Overcoming Resentment and Anger
Volume 41: Resolving Blockages and Positive Thinking
Volume 42: Stress Reduction, Stress Management
Volume 43: Body Relaxation
Volume 44: Deep Relaxation
Volume 45: Fear of the Dark
Volume 46: Falling Asleep and Staying Asleep
Volume 47: Compulsive Buying
Volume 48: Restless Legs Syndrome
Volume 49: Bulimia
Volume 50: Anorexia
Volume 51: Overcoming Nightmares
Volume 52: Imagined Deformity
Volume 53: Overcoming Distrust, Finding Trust
Volume 54: Processing Failures
Volume 55: Humiliation, Emotional Hurt
Volume 56: Distressing Compassion, Vicarious Suffering
Volume 57: Self-Forgiveness
Volume 58: Self-Awareness, Self-Confidence
Volume 59: Saying No
Volume 60: Assertiveness
Volume 61: Setting Boundaries and Self-Assertion
Volume 62: Decision-Making Ability

Volume 63: Success Orientation
Volume 64: Ruminating, Circular Thinking
Volume 65: Accepting Pregnancy
Volume 66: Birth Preparation
Volume 67: Spiritual Opening
Volume 68: Joy of Life and Inner Lightness
Volume 69: Patience and Inner Peace
Volume 70: Fibromyalgia and Rheumatism
Volume 71: Irritable Bowel Syndrome, Crohn's Disease
Volume 72: Fear of Nausea, Emetophobia
Volume 73: Stuttering and Cluttering, Speech Flow Disorders
Volume 74: Concentration and Knowledge Anchoring
Volume 75: Vitality and Spontaneity
Volume 76: Searching for Meaning and Finding Goals
Volume 77: Life Crises, Life Events
Volume 78: Workaholism, Goal Obsession
Volume 79: Helper Syndrome, Helpless Helpers
Volume 80: Medication Abuse
Volume 81: Gambling Addiction
Volume 82: Internet Addiction, Smartphone Addiction
Volume 83: Hoarding Disorder, Compulsive Collecting
Volume 84: Conspiracy Thoughts, Overvalued Ideas
Volume 85: Fear of Operations and Treatments
Volume 86: Fear of Aging
Volume 87: Travel Anxiety
Volume 88: Anxiety When Urinating, Paruresis
Volume 89: Fear of Intimacy and Togetherness
Volume 90: Fear of Blushing
Volume 91: Coming Out in Homosexuality
Volume 92: Charisma Training
Volume 93: Migraines and Chronic Headaches
Volume 94: Overcoming Allergies, Bronchial Asthma

Volume 95: Normalizing Blood Pressure
Volume 96: Compulsive Perfectionism
Volume 97: Sports Hypnosis, Motivation
Volume 98: Sports Hypnosis, Performance Enhancement
Volume 99: Determination and Focus
Volume 100: Encountering the Inner Child
Volume 101: Cravings, Binge Eating
Volume 102: Stimulating Metabolism
Volume 103: Bipolar Mood Swings
Volume 104: Borderline, Identity Crises
Volume 105: Hypomania, Euphoria, Mania
Volume 106: Restlessness, Agitation
Volume 107: Nervous Breakdown
Volume 108: Adjustment Disorders
Volume 109: Self-Alienation, Depersonalization
Volume 110: Ending Self-Pity
Volume 111: Primary Gain of Illness
Volume 112: Secondary Gain of Illness
Volume 113: Bullying, Victim Support
Volume 114: Letting Go of Envy and Jealousy
Volume 115: Fear of Spiders, Arachnophobia
Volume 116: Fear of Dogs or Cats
Volume 117: Fear of Strangers, Xenophobia
Volume 118: Excessive Worries, Generalized Anxiety
Volume 119: Strengthening Sense of Responsibility
Volume 120: Unrequited Love, Heartache
Volume 121: Work-Life Balance
Volume 122: Letting Go of Unattainable Goals
Volume 123: Allowing and Accepting Help
Volume 124: Letting Go of Adult Children
Volume 125: Tourette Syndrome
Volume 126: Life Changes and New Starts

Volume 127: Accepting Life in a Wheelchair
Volume 128: Understanding and Overcoming Homesickness
Volume 129: Understanding and Overcoming Wanderlust
Volume 130: Dizziness, Meniere's Disease
Volume 131: Overcoming Aggression
Volume 132: Cutting and Self-Harm
Volume 133: Hair Pulling, Trichotillomania
Volume 134: Postpartum Depression
Volume 135: For Relatives of Dementia Patients
Volume 136: Self-Harm, Artificial Disorders
Volume 137: Activating Self-Healing Powers
Volume 138: Preventing Depression Relapse
Volume 139: Reactive Psychoses, Follow-Up
Volume 140: Obsessive Thoughts and Impulses
Volume 141: Compulsive Checking
Volume 142: Compulsive Counting, Symmetry Obsession
Volume 143: Compulsive Washing, Cleanliness Obsession
Volume 144: Compulsive Questioning
Volume 145: Dissociative Paralysis
Volume 146: Phantom Pain
Volume 147: Overcoming Complaining
Volume 148: Hay Fever, Pollen Allergy
Volume 149: Sexual Abuse, Victim Support
Volume 150: Standing Strong Against Sexism, #metoo
Volume 151: Binge Eating
Volume 152: Overcoming Thoughts of Revenge
Volume 153: Detachment from the Aggressor, Stockholm Syndrome
Volume 154: Courage to Separate
Volume 155: Chronic Fatigue, Exhaustion
Volume 156: Fear of the Future, Existential Anxiety
Volume 157: Excessive Worry About Children
Volume 158: Fear of Failure

Volume 159: Ending Distrust and Control
Volume 160: Dejection, Dysphoria
Volume 161: Boreout, Chronic Boredom
Volume 162: Bipolar Disorders, Relapse Prevention
Volume 163: Mania, Relapse Prevention
Volume 164: Nihilism, Feelings of Worthlessness
Volume 165: Thumb Sucking
Volume 166: Being Brave
Volume 167: Being Proud
Volume 168: Overcoming Shyness
Volume 169: Being Able to Delegate Responsibility
Volume 170: Being Able to Show Emotions
Volume 171: Letting Go of Guilt, Victim Support
Volume 172: Processing Guilt, Offender Support
Volume 173: Mood Swings, Cyclothymia
Volume 174: Lack of Drive, Vital Sadness
Volume 175: Hearing Voices with Reality Reference
Volume 176: Confident Communication
Volume 177: Standing Up for Oneself
Volume 178: Taking New Paths
Volume 179: Confident Job Application
Volume 180: No Longer Being Taken Advantage Of
Volume 181: End of Submissiveness
Volume 182: Depressive Numbness
Volume 183: Mood Drops, Affective Incontinence
Volume 184: Mood Instability
Volume 185: Somatoform Disorders
Volume 186: Stomach Ulcer, Psychosomatic
Volume 187: Accepting Amputation
Volume 188: Overcoming and Letting Go of Hatred
Volume 189: Ending Accusations
Volume 190: Allowing Tears, Being Able to Cry

Volume 191: Finding and Sorting Repressed Feelings
Volume 192: Somatoform Pain
Volume 193: Living Autonomously
Volume 194: Anhedonia, Joylessness
Volume 195: Persistent Sadness
Volume 196: Obesity, Food Addiction
Volume 197: Parents of Abused Children
Volume 198: Letting Go and Letting Be
Volume 199: Childhood Sexual Abuse
Volume 200: Fear of Loss

www.ingramcontent.com/pod-product-compliance
Lightning Source LLC
Chambersburg PA
CBHW030459220526
45464CB00006B/2582